Partnering with Patients

The "art" of heart failure management

By

Nancy Spring Bartholomew, MN, NP

INFINITY
PUBLISHING

ISBN 978-0-7414-8486-4

Printed in the United States of America

Published April 2013

INFINITY PUBLISHING
1094 New DeHaven Street, Suite 100
West Conshohocken, PA 19428-2713
Toll-free (877) BUY BOOK
Local Phone (610) 941-9999
Fax (610) 941-9959
Info@buybooksontheweb.com
www.buybooksontheweb.com

Table of Contents

Dedication 5

Why I Wrote This Book 7

Foreword 9

Reflections/Purpose 11

Stories

An Unnecessary Death 13

New Orleans Transplant 17

A Team Effort 22

Frequent Flyer 26

Raised in Ethiopia 31

"Just Shoot Me!" 34

A Tough Pair of Norwegians 37

A Bundle of Energy 40

Tears of Joy 43

A Hermit No More 45

A Scared Young Man 48

The Wonders of Medication 50

Flirty Berty 54

A Gentle Muslim Man 56

The Jokester 58

"I have slimmed down" 60

"I thought you could make me feel better" 63

You are late!!!! 68

Attitude 72

An Independent Couple 76

A Tiny Strength 81

A Gentle Giant 86

A Political Dynamo 90

Performance Outcomes 93

Patient Improvements 105

Dedication

The book is dedicated, first and foremost, to the patients and their families who were cared for at the Cardiac Enhancement Center. They gave me great joy.

The caring staff deserve all the gratitude I can heap in their direction; thanks Lauri, Katy, Ruth, Randi & Sam. You helped create the environment that made patients feel cared about and welcome. The Heart Failure Team, especially the Heart Failure Resource Nurses, provided invaluable care for patients and their families...thanks Kathy & team!

A special thank you to Steve Brown for his vision, positive attitude, leadership, and encouragement.

A sincere thank you to Mark Vossler for his knowledge of heart failure management, his acceptance, and support.

Always in love, support and encouragement my deep appreciation goes to my husband, David and the rest of my loving family. Extra hugs for Michelle, for sharing her excellence in editing.

Why I Wrote This Book

Through the years, many have encouraged me to write articles to share with others some of the techniques for successful heart failure management. After mulling this over, I reflected on the reasons why I enjoy what I do…the patients! Partnering with patients, especially those with serious health problems and multiple behavioral issues, has proven to be fulfilling, rewarding, challenging and effective…so I wanted to share some of their stories to demonstrate the "art" of heart failure management. The science of evidence-based medicine is well covered by others. So these stories reflect the art of medicine, or how to manage patients within their preferences, idiosyncrasies, likes, dislikes, and cultural barriers. Basically, I used the "art" of heart failure management to get to the evidence-based science in the treatment of patients. Names have been changed, and some details added or omitted, to protect confidentiality. Along the way, I have laughed, cried, hugged, and enjoyed patients and their loved ones. I have also been frustrated, hurt and upset by them. It has overall been a joyful and enriching experience, as well as an honor to feel the trust, friendship, and love of those I have cared for over the years.

Foreword

The science of heart failure management using evidence-based treatment is well published and understood. It is utilized throughout the country and in most parts of the world, and is quite standardized. It is the "art" of heart failure management that is the finesse of management; how you come alongside of patients to get them to participate in the evidence-based treatment. The most successful providers and centers are those who utilize the combination of the "art" and the science; basically partnering with patients in moving them towards improved health. It is coming alongside of them, identifying barriers holding them back or slowing them down, and helping to overcome these barriers.

The barriers are many, including emotional, financial, cultural, and many other factors. It can be as simple as providing transportation for a patient to get to the center; or as complex as overcoming an unsupportive, abusive home situation. The barriers can be anything that interferes with the ability of a patient or loved one to monitor and care for the disease state. This is routinely called self-management or home management, and it is essential in any chronic disease. This is the day to day monitoring and care to keep the disease stable or to improve it. It includes taking medications consistently, food preparation and eating, monitoring of daily weight and other signs and symptoms, and then reporting them as necessary.

Reflections/Purpose

Our health care system in America is broken. There is fragmented care, with poor communication between those caring for patients. Most of the electronic medical records are not linked together, so there are multiple systems that do not "talk" to one another. This creates frustration for patients who are asked time and time again to repeat their story, and to list their medications and past health history. Sometimes in a new hospitalization, a patient is asked to repeat it multiple times the same day, first to the emergency room doctor, then to the admitting nurse, then to the admitting doctor, and then to specialists asked to help care for the patient. If the patient was not ill and exhausted before the hospitalization, they certainly will be moved in that direction with all the redundant questions!

Indicative of this problem is the seemingly simple question of "What medications are you taking?" Does this mean what is actually prescribed or the schedule and routine that fits in best with the patient's lifestyle? Does it include the over-the-counter medications, potions, and remedies? Does it include the number and names of prescribers of the medications? How about the reasons the patient is taking them... or not taking them?

Studies show that errors with medications are very common. They lead to unnecessary hospitalizations, complications during the hospitalization, and re-admissions to the hospital after discharge. This is particularly true with heart failure management because of the complexity of the medications and the common co-existing health problems.

However, despite the brokenness of the current healthcare delivery system, there are many who are involved in a care model that is patient-centered. By this I mean the type of care that puts the patient's care and comfort as the major focus; patient care that creates a system that strives to move patients to optimal wellness, within the limits of their disease state. This is the type of care I worked hard at delivering, usually with success, but there were failures. Some of the stories will be shared here, in the hope that others can learn from stories about partnering with patients, and demonstrations of the "art" of heart failure management.

This book is written in two voices. The first will be explanatory in nature, citing the concept or point being made. The second is the story that illustrates partnering with patients.

Ego versus Others

The practice of medicine can be intoxicating. The mere fact that lives are in the healthcare workers' hands can swell egos. If it stopped there, that would be fine. But egos can and do negatively impact patient care as this story illustrates.

An Unnecessary Death

Many years of my nursing profession were spent working in critical care at a major metropolitan hospital. Almost three decades ago, I was working the evening shift. We cared for patients who were critically ill with medical conditions like heart attacks as well as in the surgical recovery time for those needing continuous monitoring. A few hours into the shift, a man returned from the recovery room after having a carotid endarectomy. The carotid is the large artery on each side of the neck that brings blood to the brain. The surgical procedure used to clear this patient's clogged carotid was to open the artery while the blood is bypassed, cut out the diseased section, then sew in a graft to increase the blood supply to the brain. It was a very effective means of improving the blood supply.

The man was quite stable with normal blood pressure and pulse. He was awake and responsive, and his supportive wife was allowed into the room. She was at first dismayed by the large white dressing on his neck, and the multiple lines and wires, but was reassured by explanations, as well as the smile and kind words from her husband.

As the evening progressed, the man became slightly restless and developed some mild respiratory effort. It was partially relieved with pain medication; however he eventually began to make some mild low-pitched noises with each inspiration. This is called strider and can be a sign of a narrowed airway. I alerted the charge nurse and called the surgeon. He was irritated with the call and said my concerns were unwarranted. At this hospital, we had residents -- or training doctors -- although they did not usually work with this surgeon. I was used to working very closely with the residents because they were frequently around with the critically ill patients on the unit, so I knew most of them quite well. I called the surgical resident who agreed to come and see the patient, although this was not the norm for a patient of this particular surgeon. He examined the patient, ordered an x-ray of the neck, and provided reassurance to the patient and me. The x-ray was not concerning, but the patient appeared to be making more effort to breathe. He wanted up in the chair, so I helped him up with all his wires and tubes, and positioned him comfortably with a pillow on his table in front of him, where he rested his head. I called the surgeon again, and he was angry that I had asked for the involvement of the surgical resident. He refused to come in to examine the patient.

I knew this was serious but did not feel there was support or backup for this man in distress. I ordered a large bore needle in case it was needed in an emergency to establish a short term airway, and taped in on the headboard of his bed. I alerted the respiratory therapist of the situation. It was late on a Friday night and my shift was ending. In my taped report I expressed concern about the man, and gave an example of the strider-type breathing he was doing. I alerted the surgical resident of my ongoing concern, I called the surgeon again (and put up with an irritable rebuke for my stupidity), and I bid a farewell to the patient and his wife. As it turns out, it was my final farewell to him. A few hours after I left, he had a respiratory arrest and was not able to breathe because of a total airway obstruction. The unexpected swelling from his incision had cut off his breathing. The surgical resident denied the strider (but fortunately I had demonstrated it to the oncoming shift on my taped report), the surgeon said he should have been told the seriousness of the situation.... and the patient died.

I was devastated because it was a preventable thing. A breathing tube could have been inserted to support the airway and prevent the obstruction. It is a vivid example of a breakdown in health care. There was a hierarchical system, with lines of communication that were not effectively responded to, with too much power at the top of the line to an indifferent and egotistical surgeon. There was massive denial on the part of the doctors: “I did not know it was that bad”, and “his breathing did not sound like that when I saw him”. The wife was told it was a complication of the surgery (of course, not due to an unresponsive doctor). Fortunately, things have improved through the years.

Years later this still haunts me, but it has also motivated me. Since that time, I have tried even harder to be an advocate for patients and their families; to partner with them in moving toward improved health; to intervene with simpler directions and instructions; to overcome my shyness and be the strong voice for the voiceless and to stand with the powerless. I try to do my small part, in my corner of the world, to provide the best care I can for patients and their families.

PsychoSocial and Non-Compliance

By definition medical practitioners are scientists. Accordingly, we tend to focus on the evidence-based science in providing care to patients. Yet we are dealing with humans, and if we fail to address the human side of their needs the science will fail us.

One of the biggest factors negatively impacting outcomes are patients who do not follow our recommendations, otherwise known as non-compliance. There are many reasons why patients do not comply. The solution is to come alongside the patient, spend time with them, provide them with ongoing explanations, and enlist the support of their loved ones.

New Orleans Transplant

One sweet, but very simple man (I will call him Willy) came to our area after the devastation in New Orleans. He had never married, lived in a tiny house, and worked nights as a janitor until he relocated to our area. He was set up in a small apartment with the help of his one relative, a niece. His symptoms started when he began to get a little breathless with carrying his small bag of groceries from the store next to his apartment, and his shoes got too tight for his feet. He altered his life a bit by taking fewer trips to the store, stopping frequently on the way to and from, and wearing looser slippers. One night he was not able to sleep because he could not get his breath, so he called his niece who called the medics. In the emergency department he was found to have severe heart failure, with an enlarged and inefficient heart that was down to 5% function. He was hospitalized for several days under the care of an excellent cardiologist, and then was referred to me for ongoing care on an outpatient basis.

During the initial patient visit, 90 minutes were allocated, and patients were encouraged to bring along their main support people. Hence Willy came with his niece. He walked slowly into the center, stopping a few times to rest and catch his breath, then was seated at a table. Explanations about the reasons he was referred were given: "You have decreased heart function, called heart failure, but it can be stabilized and improved. Our goal is to help you feel better, and keep you out of the hospital." That usually gets their undivided attention... and it is followed by education about heart failure management. This includes instruction about things that need to be monitored and why (like daily weight, shortness of breath and swelling); education about their diet (low salt and to limit their intake of fluid); the importance and actions of the essential medications; as well as activity guidelines and emotional responses.

It is not uncommon to have patients and their family express fear, anxiety, depression, and hopelessness. Many tears are shed during this initial visit. Patients usually have not been feeling well for quite a long time, they are scared from their hospitalization and new diagnosis, a bit overwhelmed, and feeling physically poor. We take this into consideration and modify the education and patient visit accordingly. With Willy, it became apparent his reading and writing were at an elementary school level. His materials and explanations had to be at his level in order for him to understand. This was done. He was given a scale, and taught how to use it. He felt he could write down his daily weight. Fortunately his niece was able to assist with the medications, so a medication kit for a week was given to her, along with a list of the medications and a schedule.

Willy was seen once a week initially. During this time, relationships and trust were building, and his medications and care were adjusted to continue his improvement. As he began to feel better and stronger, he was pleased that he was now able to do some of the things he enjoyed. He was able to walk to the store daily, and could go to church on the days he was able to get a ride with another member. His niece continued to assist with his medications, and he took them as prescribed. He was unwilling and unable to make dietary changes because he loved sausages and other high salt foods. We adjusted his meds accordingly and had him keep track of signs and symptoms of holding on to extra fluid (with his weight going up and being short of breath and swelling in his legs and belly).

After several months he was feeling much better, and his cardiologist repeated an evaluation of his heart that showed an improvement in function, now up to 30%. He was moving in the right direction! With this good news, the frequency of his visits to the center decreased initially to every 2 weeks, then to once a month. He was stable for over a year, then began to have a return of symptoms. The cardiologist increased his water pill, and we increased the frequency of his visits to our center. He did not seem to be feeling any better with the change in meds, so after a few weeks I attempted to determine causal factors. He sheepishly admitted that he was not taking his water pills, and would pull them out of the med sets his niece was setting up for him. He did not like the urgency of urination, and had some embarrassing moments on the bus and in church.

After listening, and showing empathy, we began to work together on a plan that would work for him. He was not averse to taking the water pills because he knew they helped him feel better, but he did not want to take them during the day. We worked out a plan for him to take them in the afternoon, when he returned from his routine errands. His niece agreed to adjust things, but did express irritation with Uncle Willy for causing problems and not following directions. His compliance improved, and he continued to do some of the things he enjoyed during the day.

In caring for Willy, I learned not to assume things. We cannot assume a patient is taking the medication we prescribe. In addition, patient safety is of utmost importance, as demonstrated by what happened one day. One day, during our clinic visit, he shared a concern about one of his pills that he did not think he would be able to take. He reached into his pocket, pulled out a handful of desiccant cylinders found in some pill containers, looked at me with his big brown eyes, and said “Dr. Nancy, I do not think I could swallow them." I took them from him gently, hugged him, and said with a smile, "You did the right thing to bring those here, because they are not pills. They help to keep your pills dry. Thank you for not taking them!" Whew, scary for me!

Willy is a heartwarming example of success with heart failure management. He improved so much that he was able to enjoy trips to the Grand Canyon, Las Vegas, Texas, and other locations to enjoy God's beautiful creation and spend time with family. We would pack up his medications carefully, with enough to last until he would return. Then he would faithfully take them, and watch daily for changes. He had no problems on any of his trips.

Teamwork

Synergy is often described as 1 + 1 = 3. Teamwork works the same way. When an individual healthcare provider works independently to assist a patient, he or she is not as successful as when the providers work together as a team. The outcomes are greater than the sum of the parts.

A Team Effort

One of the problems with health care is silos – where individual organizational units hold information yet don't share that information with parallel organizational unit. This results in inefficiencies and reduces cooperation and communication between them. One of the ways we overcame this was to formulate a Heart Failure Team. We met monthly in an action-packed, efficient hour, dealing with issues of heart failure management throughout the continuum. We included three patient representatives on this team as well as professionals from all phases of care. This included the emergency department, critical care, telemetry, palliative and hospice care, our hospital-based call center, the local senior center, and the largest skilled nursing facility in the area. This was truly a multidisciplinary team approach, which was essential in dealing with the various topics to improve patient care.

This team was extremely helpful in dealing with problem patients. One patient in particular was causing me frustration and the group came up with solutions to improve the management. I will call her Susan, a woman in her 40s who was divorced and trying to raise a rebellious 15 year old. Susan had an enlarged, inefficient heart due to a familial cardiomyopathy. She had had several cardiac arrests, when her heart would pump erratically, and she had some memory issues related to a lack of blood to her brain during some of those times. The initial frustration for me came when she would sweetly make appointments to come in for her initial visit to the center, and time after time not show up. That resulted in a 90 minute empty slot in the schedule that could have been filled by another patient if we had known. After 5 or 6 times of her not showing up for appointments, I called her cardiologist and apologized that it did not seem to be working out for us to manage her heart failure because we could not get her into the center, so I was not going to call her again. He said "Please, please call her again, and do whatever is needed. She REALLY needs your care!" Then he told me more about Susan, and I began to formulate a plan. We had a call center at the hospital and part of it included some dedicated nurses who focused on heart failure. They met patients in the hospital, initiated education, evaluated for needs after discharge, and did follow up phone calls for a month to reinforce teaching as well as evaluate problem areas. I asked if they would be willing to call Susan the night before, as well as the morning of the appointment, and even an hour before the appointment. They willingly made the reminders. I also contacted the volunteer office because they had a group of dedicated volunteer drivers. Susan shared that a lack of transportation was one of the issues that kept her from coming.

With the help from these team members, Susan made it to her first appointment. She was very sweet, and tried hard to understand and please. The written materials and essential information were highlighted, and sent home with her for ongoing reminders. It was apparent that remembering to take her medications was a challenge, so we decided to take over putting them in a mediset for her. The call center nurses said they would be happy to give daily reminder calls. Susan liked the friendly reminders, and willingly participated in taking her medications as prescribed.

As her trust in us grew, she tearfully shared some of her concern about raising a rebellious 15 year-old. He was not going to school, and was taking drugs and drinking. Susan tried to be firm and consistent, but this was an ongoing battle, and she had her own lack of memory and health concerns. One of our team members was a social worker, experienced with difficulties like this, and was aware of some of the resources available. She got involved, and the son was greatly assisted by the involvement of his grandparents and a weekly counselor.

When Susan developed increasing problems with fluid retention, despite taking her medications, a further exploration of her eating revealed that she was getting much of her food at a local food bank and daily at a fast food restaurant. The team member nutritionist was alerted, and was able to come to the center during one of Susan's visits. This was very helpful in giving Susan better choices within her financial constraints. We were also able to give her volunteer driver a bag full of healthy food for a starter.

With the assistance of the team for phone call reminders, reinforcement of home management skills, transportation, medication, counseling, and nutrition, in addition to her cardiologist and nurse practitioner visits, Susan lived relatively symptom free for years. She was very sweet and appreciative, and began to think of the team members as friends. Truly her care could not have been done by one person. The teamwork was essential.

Custom Care

Many patients, especially heart failure patients, have very complicated illnesses. They require more intense attention albeit on an outpatient basis.

This intensity takes the form of frequent visits – at least at first – as well as considerable education. Additionally, systems of self-care that truly work for that individual are necessary.

Frequent Flyer

Don went into the emergency room at least once a month. He was not a hypochondriac, he just happened to have very unstable heart failure where his lungs would fill up with fluid in a matter of minutes and he could not breathe. Usually he walked into the emergency room with shortness of breath, but soon deteriorated to the point of needing a breathing tube inserted and a quick transfer to the critical care unit on life support. Fortunately, he recovered quickly, and was able to go home in a few days.

He was a divorced, 55 year old engineer. He was referred to the Cardiac Enhancement Center after a long and complicated heart surgery, where he had bypass blood vessels added to increase the supply to his heart. His cardiologist hoped that his heart would improve after bypass surgery, and that he would stay out of the hospital for longer than a month at a time. He was not able to make it in to the center for 3 weeks because he was recovering, and when he did his elderly mother wheeled him into the center in a wheelchair. He was hugging a pillow, and was scared to death! I urged him to get up from the wheelchair, taught him the correct way to transfer to the bed, and to position himself into bed. We practiced several times, until he seemed to have a feel for it, and gained some confidence in transferring independently.

Teaching him needed to be gentle, simple, and was increased at each visit to the center. He was too overwhelmed and scared to have much information retained during the first visit. In contrast, his supportive mother was thrilled to have someone else help out. Reassurance that he was improving, that he needed to move, eat and take his medications was about all that could be done at the first visit. As far as a medication adjustment, I increased his diuretic because he was holding on to too much fluid. His mother was preparing his meals, so information about healthier eating and limitation of salt was provided for her.

Initially, Don was seen weekly. He needed the frequent monitoring, and benefitted from the TLC. He was eating healthier and walking 5 minutes three times a day after a few weeks.... a big improvement. A slow adjustment of his medications began, usually every few weeks, in order to optimize the medications shown to improve heart function. He said he was taking them consistently; however sometimes his appointments would be in the afternoon and he admitted to not taking his morning meds that day. When this was explored, he said his life was a bit disorganized, and he was instructed in a system to take them that he said he would do. Shortly thereafter he ended up in the hospital… could not breathe, with fluid filled lungs and on life support. After he was discharged, we explored some of the causal factors leading to his hospitalization. He had eaten fish and chips at a local seafood restaurant, and had not taken his water pill for 2 days because he forgot. Fortunately, he was very motivated to stay out of the hospital, so we worked together to try to prevent it. Eventually, he began to see the effect salt had on his health, and he consistently started to weigh himself every morning. He saw his weight increase when he ate salty things, especially when he did not take his water pill. We worked together on a rescue plan for him to take an extra water pill when his weight was up, or he had a salty meal. We added nitroglycerine under his tongue if he had any shortness of breath with this. This small little pill is very effective in decreasing the workload of the heart, and lowering the pressures that increase when there is too much fluid in the body. This worked for many months, and he stayed out of the hospital.

One of the things that can cause, or worsen, heart failure is sleep apnea. This is a chronic medical condition where a person repeatedly stops breathing during sleep. It is very common in heart failure, and part of the routine at the initial visit is a short screening to evaluate the risks an individual has for sleep apnea. A referral to a sleep center is recommended if the screening indicates likelihood for it, so it can be diagnosed and treated. Most people feel much improved after their sleep apnea is treated, with less fatigue and increased energy.

Don was at high risk for sleep apnea, but he refused for a few years to have a sleep study. He always had various excuses, and it got to the point that I had to be quite firm with him. He eventually agreed and had a sleep study which showed severe sleep apnea. We then worked together to set up a schedule to get him accustomed to using CPAP, the positive pressure mask worn at night. It helped with his daytime fatigue.

As time went on, and the days got shorter with winter creeping around the corner, Don's impeccable grooming deteriorated. Instead of coming to the center with a crisp dress shirt, tie and nice slacks, he showed up in sweats with a few days growth of stubble. He shared that he was eating more, not going to his exercise class, and sleeping during the day. A quick depression screen showed he was depressed. This was discussed, and non-medicinal ways to improve it were covered, including daily outdoor exercise, healthier eating, and daily positive input. He was willing to incorporate these, but he was also started an antidepressant. People with chronic disease, like heart failure, have a high incidence of depression. If undiagnosed and untreated, it can interfere with home self-management, so it increases the incidence of hospitalization and death. He started the changes, including the medication, and by his next visit to the center he was back to his former self. He was also very appreciative!

Eventually his medication routine became too complicated for him to follow. This caused increased symptoms, and a few hospitalizations because of noncompliance. When this was identified as an area that needed addressing, we devised a plan. On his visits to the center, he would bring in his medications, along with medication sets. Organizing his medications would be incorporated into the patient visits. I was able to organize them as he talked about his symptoms and other things we would normally discuss at each visit to the center. With this extra help, he gave assurance that he would take them routinely; and he certainly did.

Gradually he improved to the point of only needing visits to the center once a month. His medications would still be organized during the patient visit. He was physically active daily, taking his meds routinely, eating healthily (except for rare exception when he would take extra medications as needed), and staying out of the hospital. With these changes he stayed out of the hospital for 4 ½ years! A BIG improvement from his emergency visits once or twice a month.

Meeting Patients Where They Are

It is a mistake to assume that patients are the same even if they have identical diagnosis. Not only is it likely their disease is different from the next person, but the patient is different from the next patient. Proper care means meeting the patient where they are. This entails understanding a broader spectrum of the factors that influence their condition. This often goes well beyond their physical assessment.

Raised in Ethiopia

Her daughter brought her into the center, desperate to find someone to manage her mother's health. The first day I met Anna, I was struck by her natural beauty, and the strong poise with which she carried herself. Raised in Ethiopia, the only daughter of Scandinavian physicians, she had bright blue eyes, high cheekbones, thick white hair, and a lovely complexion for a woman in her mid-80s. She was resistant to health care, terrified of doctors, and fiercely independent, but in need of care with heart function greatly decreased from years of untreated high blood pressure.

She was very bright, but quite suspicious of any care and suggestions. She also had mild dementia. I had to tread gently and lightly, first to gain her trust and then to attempt to find solutions she could accept. She was very well educated and loved Ethiopia; she became animated when sharing stories about the people, food and culture. She had led a very interesting life, but sometimes a veil of darkness would drop over her and she became fearful and closed off. She did not like to be touched, and taking her blood pressure, listening to her heart and lungs with my stethoscope or anything with physical contact took patience and gentleness. As she opened up after many months of visits to the center, she shared some hints of harshness and abuse at the hands of her cruel and sadistic physician parents.

In order to improve her health, her blood pressure needed to be controlled. Hospitalizations had occurred when she would develop extreme breathlessness, as her lungs would fill up with fluid because of her heart working so hard, with pressures like 240/130. In dealing with her suspicious nature and distrust of healthcare, I wanted to make medication choices that were simple, long acting, and effective for her blood pressure control, fluid balance, and heart improvement. Instead of the usual adjustment consisting of initiation of the medications, with gradual titration, I started with the higher doses that I thought would be effective. Her daughter, who came to all the visits and was an advocate in her care, called them her "heart vitamins", so I caught on and continued with this theme. It proved effective, because she took them faithfully, brought her blood pressure down to a more reasonable 135/85, and she stayed out of the hospital.

She always charmed me with her twinkling eyes and bright, but mischievous smile. I enjoyed her visits to the center, however challenging they were, because she shared interesting stories of her beloved homeland, Ethiopia.

Healthcare Providers are People too

We are skilled, trained, and experienced, and yet we are still human. We care about our patients and often become emotionally attached. The sad fact of the matter is that, working with heart failure patients, many people die while still going to the clinic, despite our best efforts. In such cases, it is very, very sad.

"Just Shoot Me!"

Whenever I prepare to see a patient, I get a mental image of them from the extensive review of the materials we obtain about their past medical history. With Barry, after looking over his health history, including a heart function of less than 10%, I had an image of an elderly, debilitated, frail man. Fifteen minutes before his initial visit to the center, in walked a handsome, confident, well-built man with a ready smile and a warm, charismatic manner. He had minimal symptoms...but a very poor heart.

As the months went on I got to know him quite well. Divorced, with three adult sons; living in a luxury condo above a nearby lake. He was retired, worked out daily at the fitness club by his home, drank a bit too much alcohol (especially given the degree of his heart failure), and had a strong social network.

He did an excellent job of monitoring his daily weight and symptoms, taking his medications as prescribed, and eating healthily; but he continued to drink 3 to 4 drinks daily. At each visit to the center his monitoring and self-care were commended, but he was strongly urged to stop his alcohol intake because of the depressant effect on the heart muscle. He was not at all amenable to giving up what he called his one last pleasure in life. I provided information, techniques, and encouragement, but then had to let it go.

Barry was very observant and sometimes would share his thoughts about some of the other patients. He was very sad and sorry for those who needed walkers, wheelchairs, and oxygen. Quietly, he would whisper, "I hope someone just shoots me if I ever get that bad," and, "Their lives must be so miserable depending on those things to live," and, "I would not live like that."

However, as the months and years went by, he began to live like that, and the odd thing was he did not seem to remember his past words. His muscle mass began to go, and his strong shoulders shrunk and his belly grew with fluid. He became fatigued, and was not able to climb stairs or walk without a walker.

After a hospitalization, one of his sons wheeled him into the center in a wheelchair, on oxygen. It almost brought tears to my eyes, as I recalled his words "Just shoot me if I ever get that bad." He was at the very point that he found so depressing, but it had been a gradual progression. His hope for improvement, his will to live, and his love of others did not fade. The adaptation of the human spirit is truly amazing. In a few months he was confined to bed on the inpatient hospice unit. Although he was too ill and weak to speak, his sparkling blue eyes and wide smile remained. As he looked at me, it was like he was communicating, "I am ready now." He died after three days. I was very sad, but I remembered his words, and his progression into acceptance.

Goals

Goals are powerful things. People use goals in many aspects of life, from athletics to business. They also play a vital role in healthcare. Research has shown that the existence of goals will change behavior, especially when they are monitored a reported.

In healthcare, the setting of goals can help the patient feel involved and in control as well as motivated and informed.

A Tough Pair of Norwegians

I met with a husband/wife team referred to the center. The husband was seen first, Bjorn; a rotund, thick-necked, ruddy cheeked, tough but tender elderly gent. He was accompanied by two of his blond-haired, blue-eyed, supportive, Americanized daughters at every visit. His daughters basically left their husbands and children for days at a time to move into their parents' home to cook, clean, and care for him and his wife, Berta. The daughters watched their parents' daily weights and other signs and symptoms, administered the meds, and reported symptoms to us several times a week.

Bjorn's heart failure stabilized after we got his blood pressure under control. He continued to have severe lung problems from his many years of smoking 3 packs a day, but fortunately he had stopped the habit three years prior. His wife was not so stable, or compliant. She was in and out of the hospital every week or two, and it took a few months before we were finally able to see Berta in the center. At the first visit in, they filled the room; Berta, Bjorn, and the two daughters who usually came with their dad were joined by a third daughter. They were all very eager to do whatever possible to stop the revolving door of hospitalizations for Berta. As her husband Bjorn talked about it, his tears broke through his blustering manner, and he said "I cannot go and see her in the hospital. I get too worried." Bertha looked quite ill; emaciated, dusky around her lips, sunken eyes, and hollow cheeks. She had smoked too many cigarettes, and too little healthy food, and now with heart failure, decreased kidney function, and chronic lung disease had taken its toll on her vitality.

Berta was willing to let her daughters cook, clean, administer her meds... but not to take away her cigarettes. She refused to give them up! Her family called her a "Stubborn Norwegian," and all were exasperated with her. As I came alongside of her and her family in her heart failure management, she shared that she was used to being very strong and independent and did not like to be told what to do. In understanding this, I worked with her on a plan for smoking cessation. She thought it would be doable to cut her smoking in half each week, and then to stop. We started a chart with dates and a plan. She liked seeing the progress, liked being in charge, and actually started feeling better, and her visits to the hospital became further and further apart. She liked that! As she returned to many of her activities she enjoyed, like cooking Norwegian specialty foods for her family, and cleaning her kitchen; her spirits soared. She loved caring for others! Her kind and generous actions were many, including her bringing candy and home baked goods to us when she came for her routine visits to the center. Her hands were never idle, and she always brought some knitting or other handiwork in with her to be productive during the short wait for her visit. Some of these became gifts, and I daily use the white cotton crocheted kitchen cloth she gave me. I think of her every time I use it.

As both Berta and Bjorn improved, their visits to the center lengthened from weekly to every 2 weeks, then every three, then once a month. Their daughters' phone calls became quite rare, and things settled into a fairly normal pattern for the family. Berta was successful in quitting smoking as well as staying out of the hospital for about a year. It was a welcome relief for her, Bjorn, and their daughters. It had been a good year; then suddenly Berta developed a severe respiratory infection, and she was not able to regain her oxygenation. Her strength, and then her life, gently faded away with all of her family by her side in the busy intensive care unit. I enjoyed caring for this loving and close-knit family.

Round Peg and Square Hole

Healthcare has evolved into a one-size-fits-all system in too many cases. But each individual is unique and their health needs to be managed in a unique way. Often, the system doesn't allow that. Take Mia in the story below. Significant portions of her health management occurred over the phone. Unfortunately, this is not a covered treatment, and so many healthcare providers cannot or will not provide this option, even when it is fully appropriate and far more cost-effective than a visit to the emergency room.

A Bundle of Energy

The first time I met Mia, she enthusiastically greeted me with a hug and a kiss. Her beautiful olive, Puerto Rican complexion went well with her brightly colored dress, matching hat, scarf and jewelry. To some, it may have seemed a bit overdone, but she flowed well with it. She was accompanied by her daughter and son-in-law, who patiently lent support and information when they could get a word in... which was not often. Mia offered a steady stream of conversation, with much inflection and passion. She was a bundle of energy, with much laughter and hand gesturing. It was a challenge to obtain the information needed, and the teaching was barely possible.

As the months cycled into years of caring for Mia, the pattern of her life changed dramatically with the seasons.

The high energy time, such as when I first met her, was followed in a few months by a time of nearly normal affect and responses, with less flamboyant dress and actions. This ebbed into a time of solitude and hibernation. During this time she rarely came into the center, rarely left her room, put on weight because of inactivity, and did not speak much.

During her high energy cycle, she ate excessively and inappropriately. For example, she would head out of her retirement home on her electric scooter, drive erratically in the street, sidewalks, and store fronts to buy whole pizzas and other high sodium foods that she rapidly engulfed. She would call into the center frequently during this time, and we would try to see her weekly in order to keep her out of the hospital. At each visit during this cycle, her voice and laughter would fill the waiting room as she entertained the other patients while she waited to see us; sometimes quite a wait because she would usually arrive at least an hour before her scheduled visit. Despite optimal outpatient management, she would get worked up in the wee hours of the morning and call the medics. They usually would take her into the emergency room, where she was well known, and not necessarily appreciated for her loud and sometimes demanding behavior and complaints.

Needless to say, establishing a routine for home management was nearly impossible. After months of difficulty, she said she would agree to assistance at her retirement home, but with some limitations. She allowed them to weigh her, monitor her blood pressure, and administer most of her medications. She maintained control of her diuretics, which was fine because she would call into the center and would discuss the situation with us, and we would meet mutual agreement with the dose and timing of her water pill. She also was resistant to taking her medications to control her diabetes, so this continued to be a discussion at each visit to the center. Eventually she understood her heart failure was easier to manage when her blood sugars were controlled; thus her willingness to take these particular pills increased.

She dramatically improved through the years, with her heart function moving from just 15% to normal. She felt better, stayed out of the hospital, improved her relationships with her family, and added much joy to my life. A lovely, effervescent woman, fun but challenging to work with!

Sometimes Things Go Right

Unfortunately, it is all too easy to focus on the problems, the failures, the deaths, or the belligerent patient. But in many cases, things go well.

In this story, things did go well. The patient was compliant, engaged, and her health improved. And, she was very sweet and appreciative.

Tears of Joy

Hui Zhong was always accompanied by her daughter and an interpreter. She understood some English, but was embarrassed to speak it in front of me. What was interesting about Chinese being interpreted is that she and the interpreter would talk for long periods of time in Chinese, and then the interpreter would say one sentence in English. I always thought I was missing out on something important! One strong message that came across was how appreciative she and her family were with the care she was receiving. The first time she shared this, she and her daughter had tears streaming down their faces as they told me about her son who had died at a young age because of inadequate health care. They said he would be alive today if only I had cared for him. Quite moving and optimistic!

Hui Zhong was so wonderful to care for, because she would receive instructions and follow them exactly. She would come in with extensive charts of her daily weights, blood pressures and symptoms; with her medication list and any changes that had been made; and with charts about how much time she spent walking every day. She was motivated to improve, and to do the best she could. Delightful!

She and her daughter would also usually come with gifts. Sometimes they were delicately decorated pastries with intricate designs they had made. Once it was a beautiful vase they brought back from the Emperors Avenues in China. Another time it was a lovely scarf, then perfectly packaged tea along with an interesting handcrafted tea mug. They were generous, appreciative, demonstrative and very motivated to stay as healthy as possible. I saw her for years, and she successfully stayed out of the hospital. It was great to have such motivation and appreciation, and I always enjoyed the diversity of dealing with people from different cultures.

One Step at a Time

It is common to have multiple health issues at the same time, especially with heart failure patients. Often some of the problems are physical and others are emotional. Yet they work together, for better or worse.

The poor health of these patients dictates the pace at which we can treat their various issues. In the case of Harold, the pace was very slow, but produced very pleasing results.

A Hermit No More

The first time I met Harold he was in dirty sweats with stringy white hair to his shoulders. He was quite a hermit and very socially awkward. As he shared his story, it became apparent that he was very bright and well educated. He said it was very difficult for him to come to the center because his wife had died of cancer a few years before in the same facility, and that coming to see me was the first time he had been back since his wife died. After he shared that information, he paused as a shadow crossed his face, and he said when he found out she had died he jumped three stories down in the hospital stairwell, was injured, and spent a month in a psychiatric hospital. After sharing this, he smiled, and said he was doing better now.

After obtaining his health history and doing some teaching, it was time to examine him. The first time I touched him, he startled and almost jumped off the table. He had not had any physical contact since his wife died. After the initial shock, he settled down and the exam was able to be completed.

Initially he was seen weekly, because he had been quite unstable and was very socially isolated. Baby steps were needed with Harold. As the weeks rolled into months, he began to open up more and more. His appearance improved. He began to dress in nice cotton shirts and slacks with belts; and he even got a haircut! He looked like a new man, and was actually quite handsome!

As his physical appearance improved, so did his disease self-management. He started to weigh daily to monitor his fluid balance, take his meds as prescribed, and eat a bit better. He would put up a barrier when daily walking was discussed. He told me he had been a professional bike racer, and it was hard for him to walk slowly when he was used to moving so fast on a bicycle. I talked with him about the benefits of a cardiac rehab program, thinking it would help with his social isolation and allow him to use a stationary bike. He demonstrated anxiety just talking about it, so a plan was made.

At each visit to the center, the benefits of cardiac rehab would be discussed. He began to appear more comfortable as time went on. Then one day, I said we would walk down and take a look at the cardiac rehab facility together. We made it to the door of the center, and then he told me he was too anxious to go further so we stopped. He was flushed, and nervous, in a full-fledged anxiety attack...but also a bit proud of himself for going that distance. Eventually we made it all the way in the door, and I introduced him. After that, he agreed to go. As it turned out, those sessions three times a week helped turn his life around. He excelled on the bikes and got in shape, made friends, (one of which became a serious lady friend), and really enjoyed himself. His new friends encouraged him to resume one of his former hobbies, fixing up race cars and racing. He was not able to race, but he restored a race car and was able to drive it around the track on non-racing days. He was even able to squeeze into his old race car uniform...quite a joy and surprise for him!

As his social isolation and mental health improved, his physical health did also. He stayed out of the hospital, and the frequency of his visits to the center lengthened from weekly, to twice a month, and then monthly. He needed that monthly contact emotionally (he called me his angel), and for accountability and disease monitoring. He would usually come in with his lady friend, who was delightful and fun. It was fun to see how far he had progressed from his initial visit to the center!

Poor Health is Not Just for the Elderly

Sometimes we see patients that are experiencing the inevitabilities of the aging process. In other cases, we see patients that are too sick for their young age because of poor lifestyle choices. But still in other cases, we see very young patients suffering primarily because of poor genes.

Some of this latter type of patient reacts to the news that they have a disease unusual for a person of their age, by totally diving in to do all they can to make the best of such a difficult situation.

A Scared Young Man

Isaac was my youngest patient. At 19, he was younger than my sons, and lived far from his mother and family in Texas. Familial Cardiomyopathy ran in his family, and his 45 year old mom had end stage heart disease. All the men in his family were drug users, and Isaac daily smoked marijuana and drank alcohol. He came to our area for work in a restaurant, and got connected with a young woman. She was great at coming along side of Isaac and moving him towards healthier choices in his life, and her family embraced this delightful young man.

At his first visit to the center, he shared his fears and loneliness. His big brown eyes filled with tears as he told how scared he was in the hospital, and how he would do anything to get better. He was a MOTIVATED LEARNER! Like a sponge he and his girlfriend listened intently to every word, taking notes and asking good questions.

During the first few months, he called several times a week to talk. Sometimes he was anxious about something he had eaten that had too much salt; sometimes he called about medication adjustments that had to be done because of side effects; sometimes to ask questions he had about his mom's health; sometimes it was relationship difficulties; sometimes it was to confess he had had some alcohol or marijuana; and sometimes I think he was just lonely and wanted a mother-like person to listen and care about him. It was hard to be a 19 year old so far from home with a chronic health condition.

After almost a year, his family sent him money to come home for the holidays. I never heard from him again. I hope and pray he is getting care for his heart failure, and is surrounded by his loving family. One can only hope...

A Book by its Cover...

It is easy to say this after the fact, but it is much harder to look past the behavior of a challenging person. By her outward behavior, Hannah was not a nice person; she was someone you didn't want to be around. However, my family and faith have taught me to love the unlovable, and usually I have found that it is something that can be accomplished. I enjoy challenges, and am usually able to look past the outward, sometimes obnoxious, behavior to the heart of the person.

Like so many of us, there was another side of Hannah, and fortunately that side came out in time for her healthcare providers to help Hannah, despite herself.

The Wonders of Medication

Her reputation preceded her. The healthcare providers expressed concern for Hannah, who had been hospitalized for 2 weeks with a new diagnosis of heart failure, and was extremely ill in critical care most of that time. They knew she would be coming to see me at the center, and they expressed concern for her well-being as well as suggested approaches they found to be most helpful. Apparently, she had been extremely difficult to manage while in the hospital, and as it turns out, one of the reasons was she had stopped her psychiatric medications. She was angry; awake all night, verbally abusive and threatening personal harm to those in her hospital room. Hence a very memorable patient, and one only the most skilled and calm healthcare providers would be assigned to care for.

There were no teachable moments during her acute illness, and the nurses assigned to initiate this teaching were somewhat frustrated. It is especially important with a new diagnosis of heart failure to provide education because the follow-up care and home management is essential for stabilization and improvement. These nurses also had the responsibility of follow-up phone calls to assess the situation at home, answer questions, and reinforce education. While in the hospital these nurses were met with Hannah tossing boxes of Kleenex or phones at them, along with angry curses. The follow-up phone calls were met with obscenities and phone slamming. They were successful however -- mostly through her supportive mother -- in making an appointment for her to be seen in the outpatient center. Soon the day arrived...

I was surprised to meet a lovely, attractive woman looking younger than her 40 years. She was accompanied by a mother who tried to be supportive, but was more interested in non-evidence based management of her heart failure using herbal potions and adrenal supplements. Hannah was bright, interested in learning, and motivated. But she was also scared. I was surprised by her pretty green eyes, creamy complexion, high cheekbones, full lips, and pretty face that was surrounded by a head of dark brown, and styled hair. One of the first things I said was "You are so pretty." She shared that she had spent many years as an international model, traveling the world in the fast-paced, competitive market of physical appearances, but was now past her prime. Her eyes teared up slightly, but did not spill over, as she shared her story of past successes and hurts. The hurts recently were a new diagnosis of heart failure, and a long, difficult, and scary time in the hospital. She asked if I had heard about some of her actions while there, and I honestly said I had. She asked me if I would please apologize to those who had cared for her, and explained she had stopped taking her psychiatric medications and had been taking illegal drugs and drinking excessive alcohol.

She was very motivated and soaked up information like a sponge. She really wanted to learn all about her disease, and wanted to do whatever possible to improve. She was a delight, because she was very bright and very motivated... indeed fear can be a good motivator.

One of the challenges in managing Hannah was her manipulative techniques. She tried to play one healthcare provider against another; and actually made up stories about some of them. I found a quick phone call to establish and maintain communication and continuity of care was essential. It was also essential she maintained routine psychiatric care at the outpatient center. If this was not stabilized, her physical health would suffer.

As the months, then years went by she did an excellent job of taking care of herself. She took her heart medication faithfully, ate healthier, avoided alcohol and illegal drugs, and walked daily. She was frustrated by the weight gain caused from her psych meds, but she felt so much better on them she was willing to live with it. Her heart function improved from 10% to normal, and she remained symptom free. I liked her, and enjoyed her, but had to be firm and consistent. It was easy to fall into her manipulative games. I also needed to protect her from her mother's potions and alternative remedies. She meant well and was doing her best, but some of the things she pushed for where not in her daughter's best interest. She also had a tendency to criticize Hannah, who was fragile and sensitive. I had to try to buffer some of that, and try to redirect Hannah's mother in pathways that were constructive and helpful. People do not live in isolation, so all of these family dynamics need to be considered in effective patient management.

We Can Only Do So Much

A person's health is the function of many variables. While it is my contention that, as healthcare providers, we need to address far more than just what medications we provide.

But there are limits. Oftentimes the patient either can't or won't be a part of the solution. The result can be very sad.

Flirty Berty

A Latino man in his mid-thirties was referred to the center for heart failure due to alcohol, called alcohol cardiomyopathy. He had been in the hospital for 15 days where he was converted out of an abnormal heart rhythm called atrial fibrillation, went through DTs and was discovered to have heart function down to 15%. He was single, a bit of a playboy, and his interactions with women were flirtatious. It was a challenge to carry on a conversation with him because he gave everything a sexual connotation. Examining him was an uncomfortable time for me because the routine taking of vital signs and listening to his heart and lungs turned into a time of pleasure for him. My usually warm, open manner would become stern and demanding, as well as cold, calculating and overly professional. It was obvious he was used to flashing his winning smile and using his charm and good looks to his advantage. I was immune. Not only was I twenty years older than him, but when I saw him it was not as an attractive hunk, but as a self-destructive alcoholic with a failing heart. He was also destructive to others because he was HIV positive and quite deceitful to his partners in his promiscuity.

Despite his flaws, he showed up consistently for his appointments to the center and seemed to be taking his medications consistently and avoiding alcohol. He stayed out of the hospital, and I was confident his heart would be improved if he continued taking better care of himself.

His pattern changed after about 6 months. He began to miss his appointments to the center and drop in at unscheduled times. I would make every attempt to fit him in because my hope was that he would improve. Usually I smelled alcohol on him, but he assured me he was taking his medications as prescribed. He used his charming techniques at every visit, but I offered firm but supportive guidance and instruction. I tried to get him set up with one of my patients who helped others overcome addictions, but Berty was not interested.

We had steady contact for a little over a year. I have no idea what happened to him, but I assume his self-destructive lifestyle got the better of him. He never seemed to learn from his mistakes, or that there are negative consequences to his actions. Our phone calls to try to arrange visits to the center were unanswered, he stopped dropping in, and then his phone line was disconnected. I would be surprised if he is still alive. It makes me sad that he never seemed to "get it" that his health could be improved.

The Downside of Partnering with Patients

The main premise of this book is that the quality and efficacy of healthcare when we, as healthcare professionals, engage with the patients in their care.

There is a downside to this, though, as this story illustrates.

A Gentle Muslim Man

Mohammad was a 60-year-old man from Iran who would always come with his adult son, who I could not understand very well because of a speech impediment on top of his language barrier. Fortunately we always had an interpreter.

His visits to the center were fun, productive and very gratifying. This man was motivated! He always came with medication lists that were in Persian and English; a daily weight chart; labs from his primary provider; and a list of questions. This helped to bridge the gap between different health care centers. He was kind, appreciative, and compliant and I always looked forward to his visits at the center. During each of his visits to the center, he would grab my hand, look at me with a smile and twinkling eyes, and say "Doctor Nancy, I like you!"

We overcame the cultural and language barrier by having excellent interpreters. We set up a schedule for his medications that worked out with his lifestyle and the medication chart we provided was translated into Persian. We discussed ways to incorporate low sodium eating into his diet. I was able to understand the explanations given for the gift of the beautiful engraved silver platter he hand carried from Iran to give me.

Then finally, the interpreter translated the farewell letter I had written to my patients and families. I was leaving to move to the mountains on the other side of the Cascade Range. As he listened, his smile faded, eyes filled with tears and he could not speak. He looked like his heart was breaking... I felt so sad. He and his son hugged me, and his son thanked me profusely. Mohammad could not speak. The interpreter, who I had gotten to know quite well over the years, hugged and thanked me also. It was hard to say goodbye... however I rest assured in knowing his health was improved and we had had a mutually enriching relationship.

Too Many Specialists; Too Many Complications

Healthcare has become a maze of silos, with islands of caregivers not communicating with each other. This can cause anxiety for the patient. They desperately want to make sense of it all, and it can be overwhelming to have numerous medical appointments with many different providers over a fairly short period of time. Helping the patient make sense of it all can be part of a comprehensive plan to address their medical needs.

The Jokester

I could always expect Rob to come to the center with at least one joke. Towards the end of his visit, he would usually start out if I had heard about.... something or other. Being ever gullible, I would seriously say, “No, tell me about it,” and he would launch into story that I would quickly figure out was a joke. He was able to keep a straight face until the end, when we would both crack up. His favorite jokes were about lawyers.

Our relationship did not start out that way. His initial visit to the center was after a prolonged hospitalization for a coronary artery bypass surgery that was complicated by kidney, lung and liver problems. He spent three weeks in the hospital and a month in a skilled nursing facility. Needless to say, his diagnosis of heart failure was only one of his multiple problems, and he had a long list of specialists. The last thing his concerned wife wanted was another provider to add to the already too complicated list. I totally understood, and took no offense. I reassured them that one of the things we worked hard at doing was coordination of care and communication with other providers. They would each be informed of every update at each visit to the center, and that most of our patients had multiple, complicated heath issues. I also explained that our goal was to make sure that the rest of his disorders were well managed, because if not, they would negatively impact heart failure management. She was skeptical on that first visit, but after the first month she gave me the vote of confidence by letting him come on his own without her!

He gradually got better and stronger. He started in a cardiac rehab program, which was excellent for him because he did not have the discipline to maintain consistent exercise on his own. His long list of medications was made more manageable when we organized it by the reason he was taking it. We worked together to devise a healthier way for him to eat (his weight had been 320 pounds for years). His diabetes improved as he became more active, and his weight gradually began to go down. His kidney function remained decreased, but stable. His heart function improved from 20% to 45%. His depression resolved. And his jokes began! I always looked forward to his visits at the center.

Motivation goes a Long Way

Sometimes healthcare workers are cheerleaders; coaxing and encouraging our patients to keep trying, to keep moving forward and making progress.

When we have a patient that is self-motivated, it often results in a corresponding health improvement.

"I have slimmed down"

The first time I met Josh I was called to another clinic to evaluate a patient they were concerned about; and rightly so. He was pale, diaphoretic, and extremely weak and lightheaded despite sitting in a wheelchair. His blood pressure was found to be 70/40, pulse 100, and oxygenation 90%. He was accompanied by his wife, a supportive, talkative, anxious woman in jeans, brightly colored sweater that clashed with her dyed red hair. She said she had given Josh all his medications at one time, and on an empty stomach, because he was on the way to see his cardiologist. We gave him some food and fluid, and kept him there until his BP was 90/ 60 and he was feeling better, and then sent him on his way.

He came to our center for an initial visit the following week. He looked much better, and was a character with a pleasant, teasing manner. He blew off his serious health problems, but his wife anxiously filled us in on the many issues he had with his health. She played a very active role in his home management, organizing his meds, cooking his meals, monitoring his weight and other signs of fluid retention. He had quit smoking and drinking because he was motivated to keep his third wife happy and involved in his life. Many years of abusing his body had taken its toll: he was on oxygen 100% of the time, and his mobility was limited by severe shortness of breath requiring a walker or wheelchair. He wanted to feel better and stronger, and to get independent enough to chop wood again.

Over the months he improved greatly. He was taking his medications 100% of the time, and we had put together a schedule that was workable for him and his wife. He was sleeping better, eating healthier, walking up to half a block per day with his walker and oxygen, and still avoiding tobacco and alcohol.

As he began to feel better, he started sharing stories of his life. He had been the mayor of the small mountain town where he lived, and still met with the "good old boys" regularly. None of them knew he stopped alcohol, and he chuckled as he told how he fooled them by drinking ginger ale on the rocks. He also enjoyed sharing some of the details of the mountain search and rescue missions he had been a part of in past years. It was as if he needed to share a time in his life when he was able to contribute more to others.

One time he happily came into the center with his walker and a jaunty gait, saying he had been working on a gradual weight loss program, and was feeling quite proud of himself.

As he stood on the scale to show me, his jeans dropped to the floor and he stood there in his brightly colored boxers. He started to laugh, as did his wife, and I joined in heartily. His wife got to laughing so hard she fell to her knees, dropped the oxygen canister she was holding, and it started rolling down the hall. When we composed ourselves, I commended him for his weight loss, as I thought to myself "I am sooo glad no other patients were in the area."

He continued to feel better, stayed out of the hospital, improved his heart function, and was able to get back to taking a few road trips. He did not get back to chopping wood, but his stepson moved in, and Josh was happy to supervise this particular chore.

The Whole Team Needs to Play

The word "team" appears countless times in this book. That is not by accident. The team approach is the ONLY way to give effective, efficient, comprehensive patient care. That team includes many healthcare professionals as well as friends and family.

But just as a sports team needs every player on the field, we need the whole healthcare team working together.

It is the patient, oftentimes, that gets to decide who is on the team and who isn't, and the basis of that decision can be emotional, not practical, as in the case with Steve.

"I thought you could make me feel better"

During a time I had allotted to paperwork catch-up, I heard a voice say, "Can you help me please?" I turned and saw a poorly groomed man in dirty clothes with a pleading look on his face. I asked him in, and sat at the table as he told me his story. He had been developing symptoms of shortness of breath and leg swelling for about a month, and found the center after reading an article about a patient who had been helped by our team. He did not have a referral, and I told him usually patients are referred to the center. His eyes teared up, and I told him I would help him today and get the referral later. I knew his doctor and he would have been fine with me seeing Steve that day. Good thing he was seen!

He was very fluid overloaded, with edema up to his knees; neck veins bulging to his jaw as he was sitting up on the examination table; fluid in his lungs that brought his oxygen saturation down to the high 80's; and a blood pressure of 190/100. He was in trouble, but he absolutely refused to go to the hospital. Good thing it was a time when there were no other patients coming in because I had my work cut out for me.

Before administering any treatment, I pulled up recent labs and hospital notes from 6 months previously. He was not on any medications and had no allergies. It was pretty urgent to begin to get rid of some fluid and to get his blood pressure down, so I administered a diuretic, potassium and then Nitroglycerine under his tongue. Within about 10 to 15 minutes his blood pressure was down to a manageable level, he was feeling better, but he REALLY needed to urinate. Fortunately, there was one close by so he sauntered over. When he returned, he was smiling and said he "peed like a racehorse," and was already feeling better. As he rested, I gave him samples of water pills, potassium and an ACE Inhibitor to lower his blood pressure and help his heart. I had an opening the next day, and he agreed to return so I could see how he was doing and draw blood work. After a few hours, and multiple trips to the bathroom to empty his bladder, he then headed straight home. After he left I called his doctor, told him what had occurred and my plan, and he was very appreciative for the help with what he called an ornery, noncompliant guy. We also discussed getting him into a cardiologist to do some tests to check the function of his heart, specifically a cardiac echo. As it turned out, I was able to schedule an echo for the same week, and an appointment with a cardiologist the following week.

When he came back the next day he was showered with clean clothes. He said he was feeling so much better! When I weighed him his weight had dropped 12 pounds! His edema was improving, neck veins were improved, and his BP was down to 142/80. His lungs were clear, and his oxygenation was in the mid-90s. At the end of the visit, he left with new prescriptions of the helpful medications, a scale, a lab slip for a blood draw, and a note showing the information for the cardiac echo and appointment for the cardiologist. He said he would weigh himself every day, take his medications as prescribed, and return early the next week for a follow up visit.

Steve looked so much better when I next saw him. As he began to improve, he was thankful but quite ornery. Many things in life would upset him and he would rant a bit at each visit to the center. Sometimes it was a line that was too long at the pharmacy; other times an issue with one of the residents at the trailer park where he helped keep up the facilities; or concerns about his grandkids, who were frequently left in his care; the confusion over the Medicare statements, or discrepancies in hospital billing. He was the treasurer at the local Gamblers Anonymous, and said he enjoyed the weekly sessions there. He would repeatedly tell me about the hazards of gambling (which was something I knew nothing about, since I had never done it), and how he had to work daily on this addiction.

He faithfully took his heart medications, and as a consequence, his heart function improved from the initial 15% function to normal. His symptoms disappeared and he became more active. Unfortunately he was diagnosed with diabetes, and refused to follow-up with an endocrinologist because he did not like him. He wanted me to continue to prescribe his medication for his diabetes, and I initially refused. Later I had to relent because he needed it and would not see anyone else, so either I did it or it did not get done. His primary care doctor was informed, and because he knew Steven quite well and knew what a challenge he was to manage, he was very supportive of my taking this on.

After a few years, his labs showed his diabetes needed improved control. When this was discussed with him, he admitted that to save money he did not take those medications consistently. It varied, but it sounded like he only took them as prescribed twice a week to stretch them out. His budget was tight, and he expected it to get tighter if his wife got laid off. As his blood sugars increased, his fluid balance became a problem again, so his heart medications and diuretics needed to be increased. Although I consistently talked with him about improving his diabetic control, he tuned me out. It was like he could not handle this one more thing! Fortunately he continued with his heart medications, and said he took them consistently.

His vision was failing, and it got to the point that he was no longer safe to drive. His visits to the center decreased in frequency, and he was only able to come in when he had a ride from someone, which was not very often. His world continued to get smaller, because he could not go to Gamblers Anonymous, the store, or the other outings. He became very depressed. His wife moved into their daughter's home because she could not deal with his criticism and depression. He sat alone, at home in his trailer, with the only one change- a weekly visit for a few hours from his grandson. He became increasingly more embittered and less compliant with his medications. I rarely saw him, and he did not answer or return the phone calls. He ended up in the hospital after many months, and was in terrible condition. His heart failure and diabetes were out of control, he was dirty and emaciated, and it looked like he may have had a stroke. When I walked into his hospital room, he started crying and said, "I wanted to call you, but I was too embarrassed." Quite pitiful, and my heart went out to him. He was a lonely man who had pushed others away. It made me quite sad.

He recovered, and was transferred to a long term facility. I was thankful because he would have consistent care, a safer environment, and social interaction. I felt sorry for the caregivers because he was not easy to be around. Not everyone is.

Love/Hate Relationship

Healthcare is a science, but it is also laden with emotion. Certainly, patients often are legitimately emotional, and sometimes, as I caregiver, I am emotional.

But that, too, is part of being in relationship with the patients – part of partnering with patients.

You are late!!!!

I am usually very timely. I hate to wait or be late for appointments so I have always tried to show the same consideration to my patients. One particular day I was running 5 to 10 minutes late because of unexpected, unusually difficult decisions for most of the patients. The new patient, Thelma, did not appreciate that I was 10 minutes past the time she was scheduled. Her first words were “I hate fucking waiting”. Wow! It was unusual to have such anger and bluntness at the initial meeting. I graciously offered my hand, apologized with a smile, and said I did not blame her, that I hated to wait also. As I led her back to the scale for weighing, then to the spacious, windowed room where we liked to do the initial visit, she mumbled that I was lucky she did not storm out. I let her vent, then started to direct the conversation towards more positive topics. I wanted to hear her story and health history before diving into the education about home management. It sounded like she had a limited support system, had a tendency to be non-compliant with medications and health care management, smoked, and loved her cat. As I observed her, I determined she was poorly groomed (obese, braless with a dirty tee-shirt and tight pants); spiked grey hair and masculine mannerisms. She was quick to anger, very blunt and direct, bright, and did not respect or trust the health care system. She did not have a primary care provider, and had only recently become involved with the cardiology team because she was extremely ill and hospitalized for many days. Hence she was here to see me on an outpatient basis. What a joy for me! NOT!

It was clear to me that she was scared to death! She was also motivated, as manifested by the fact that she was sitting before me. It was also clear that any changes needed to be SLOW, and that I needed to work very hard to build a relationship and trust with her. Also that I had to do my best to see her at exactly the time she was scheduled!

We made steady progress, but with baby steps. For every medication change or titration, she usually required three visits to convince her of the need. It was a bit frustrating, because her blood pressure usually was about 170/ to 190/; and I was very eager to get it down to the 120/ to 130/ range. Finally, after many months she was optimized on her medications, eating better, and her blood pressure and weight were stabilized. Now was the time to work on cutting down her smoking.

Over the months she began to share small bits of her life, and cautious snippets of information. She had had an abusive upbringing, did not like or trust men, loved her cat, and had a small circle of friends she enjoyed gambling with at visits to nearby casinos. As it turned out, she was addicted to gambling. She told me of one time she received an unexpected amount of money back from a tax return, and the day and night she received it she did not sleep. She was consumed... with sweaty palms, anxiety and constant thoughts of gambling to spend that small amount of cash. A few weeks later she sought out help, and began to see a counselor weekly through Gamblers Anonymous. It was quite an eye opener to me, since I had never been exposed to anything like that before.

It was very difficult to cope with her visits to the center. She was brash and outspoken, and seemed to have an attraction to me. It was like she always was trying to see how far she could push my patience. At one visit, when her blood pressure was 184/96 and blood sugar 320, and it was apparent she was not taking all of her medications as prescribed, I asked in frustration "Thelma, I cannot understand why you come to the center to see me, when you do not follow the instructions and treatment plan I recommend?" She immediately responded "Because I like you, and trust you. It just takes me awhile to change." But for the most part, I maintained calm, firm, but kind and affirming in my approach with her. I could see the scared little girl behind her gruff, obnoxious façade. Also I made sure I was never late... one minute late and she would begin to act out.

But she improved. She cut her smoking to 3 cigarettes a day, which was a big improvement from her 3 packs a day. She took her medications most of the time. Her blood pressure was controlled. We had another challenge when I had to break the news that she had diabetes and needed a primary care provider to manage it. It took about 3 months before she agreed to see someone, and to take oral medications for it. She was quite neurotic about anything new, but finally she saw a physician she liked that was closer to her home. She began to trust him to take over some of her care. Was I ever relieved! Eventually, with improvements in how she was feeling, she transferred all of her care to that physician and made the decision to not see me anymore. It was affirming, and I thought the time was good for that, as long as she continued in the positive directions she was heading. I shared that I would be available for her if she needed me, but that I felt confident she had moved in a healthier path, and was doing much better. I was actually relieved to not have to endure the battles that occurred with each visit to the center, but also quite gratified at the progress that had been made.

Bad Luck Doesn't Have to Result in "Why Me?"

Some of us do all the right things to contribute to a healthy life, but bad genes can frustrate those efforts.

When poor health results in spite of a healthy lifestyle, a bitter response is not the only possible reaction.

Attitude

A genetic predisposition to get a disease is one of the most frustrating things in healthcare for me. Some people take excellent care of themselves, and develop severe disease states; while others abuse their bodies and continue disease-free. Danny was one of those who were born with a set of unhealthy genes...

When I met him in his early 40s, I immediately liked him. He was personable, with bright laughing eyes, curly dark hair and a big smile. He was friendly, bright, hardworking...and very ill. He had had a myocardial infarction and coronary artery bypass surgery the previous year, and at that time had also been diagnosed with severe high blood pressure and diabetes. Those two diseases had likely been part of his life for many years, but he had not been seeing doctors until the year of his heart disease. His kidneys had been quite severely damaged from the untreated high blood pressure and diabetes. He had been told that he would be on dialysis within a year. He also had recently been diagnosed with heart failure.

Despite his multitude of health problems, he continued to work daily as a construction supervisor at a major metropolitan hospital. He loved his job, and had built up a great team of workers. It was better than his home life; his wife had divorced him last year when he started to develop all his health problems. A sad reality is that this situation is all too common. But Danny did the best he could, took his medications fairly consistently, ate healthily but not regular meals, and did not smoke or drink alcohol. And he maintained a great attitude! Very positive!

Over the next year or two he improved and readily incorporated the medication and eating changes made for his heart failure management. I talked to the nearby university hospital nephrologist and got Danny started along the pathway towards kidney transplant. It was quite a long and labor intensive process, and he needed encouragement to continue along and progress down this path. He had started kidney dialysis twice a week and adjusted his work schedule to accommodate this. I am sure he was fatigued all the time, but he never complained. Until one night...

After a normal, uneventful day at work, he went home to his normal routine, but during the night he had a stroke. Living alone, he was unable to move to call for help, and was not discovered until the next day around noon. His team at work was concerned when he did not show up or call, which was highly unusual for Danny. He was always prompt, ready to dive into work, and was the organizer and encourager. One of his friends from work called his landlady, explained the situation, and she went to his apartment. Immediately she called the medics, and he was taken to the hospital. Unfortunately, too much time had passed for him to receive the brain restoring treatment to save the function that had been interfered with due to the lack of blood supply. He was unable to move one of his sides, and he had a decreased ability to speak and think.

I did not see him during this phase because he was in a different hospital and I didn't even know about his stroke and hospitalization. Apparently he stayed at the hospital for rehabilitation after his stroke, went to a skilled nursing facility, and then home in the care of his elderly aunt. I found out about all of this when I called to inquire how he was doing, since he had not been seen in the center for over three months. After identifying myself on the phone, he blurted out "Nancy, I had a stroke!" I felt as though someone had kicked me in the stomach, my eyes filled with tears, and I was speechless. This gave him time to explain to me what had happened, and the progress he had made. His speech had mostly returned, although I noticed he hesitated a bit with some words. He was not able to move one of his sides, but had an electric wheelchair so he was able to get around. Everything he did took extreme effort. He was working on setting up transportation, and said he would get into the center as soon as he could. He sounded a bit overwhelmed and discouraged, but was hopeful things would get better.

When I saw him in the center a few weeks later, he wheeled in, with excellent maneuvering using his electric wheelchair. His warm smile and laughing eyes were there, but with a sadness not seen previously. During the visit, he shared his loneliness; because only one friend remained true for weekly visits... the rest had fallen to the wayside. This was difficult for a gregarious guy, who was used to leading a team, getting respect and affirmation daily. His caregiver aunt caused some concern for him because she tried to boss him around and take charge of doing some things he could do, albeit slower, but it was important for him to maintain some independence. Surprisingly enough, he really enjoyed his twice weekly dialysis sessions because he liked the routine and the socialization. He really missed his work.

But his attitude continued to be positive. Even this stroke, on top of everything else, did not keep him down long. He was arranging time for swimming twice weekly at a local handicapped friendly pool. He had set a goal to walk 5 feet into the door of his church, and had a physical therapist to help him work towards that goal. He was adjusting to the losses and changes in his life, and making the best of a horrible situation. I admired him, learned from him, and enjoyed him. He never whined, never said "Why me?;" he took a negative situation and worked hard to make something positive out of it. What a remarkable guy.

Spouses: A Vital Part of the Health Equation

Clearly, teamwork is a key to successful healthcare. A spouse or significant other can be an important and vital player on that team.

In this story, the degree to which a couple can provide mutual support is exemplified.

I try hard to include family in the healthcare equation, but in this example, it was particularly touching how they each had unique needs that the other could meet.

An Independent Couple

I met Dottie and Bud after she had been hospitalized for a few weeks, and then moved to a skilled nursing facility for a month for hypertensive heat disease, diastolic heart failure and a stroke.

They arrived together; she was a cute, white haired woman with a big smile, using a walker because of limited movement on one side since her stroke, as well as a hip that caused constant pain and was likely in need of replacement. Bud was a thin, fast moving, inpatient man who was quite doting towards his wife in his own way. He had a difficult time expressing himself, with a stuttered speech pattern and frequent inappropriate words; but between his hand motions and his wife's translations, he was able to get his point across most of the time.

Despite their deficits, they were a pretty good team. They were also similar in wanting to be as independent as possible. Both had had a very hard time during Dottie's health crisis and stay away from home. They were interested in seeing what I could do to help in their shared goal of staying at home and being as healthy as possible.

Several issues were of concern and needed to be remedied. One of the most important was his inability to assist her with taking her medications. She was not able to do it herself, and he seemed to be unable to grasp the organization of her many pills. Fortunately they agreed to have us help. Initially we set up weekly visits to the center where we could manage her care and set up her med sets at the same visit. They were thrilled with this idea, and it worked out very well.

Another area of necessity was healthier eating. Dottie had been the shopper and food preparer, but was now unable to participate in that, except in delegation. Bud did not like to be told how to do things, so he was irritable with her instructions in the kitchen. He thought canned soup and hot dogs would be fine for her, since it worked out ok for him. Unfortunately, the sodium content in what he was preparing would have sent her on a pathway back to the hospital. When they were made aware of this, both were motivated for change. A shopping list was prepared for them of healthy, low sodium, easy to prepare foods to get them started. We also met with the hospital social worker that helped to fill out the paperwork to get them started on Meals on Wheels. They have low sodium choices, which I have been told are quite tasty. After the meals started arriving, both Bud and Dottie shared with me how much they enjoyed them. That problem was solved!

As time continued on, I became concerned about Dottie's safety at home. It sounded like they had a cluttered, dirty home. Dottie had been the one in their years together who had cleaned, de-cluttered, and basically kept the home running smoothly and presentable. Now she was unable to continue this, and Bud's housekeeping skills left much to be desired. They did not want to hire someone to come in and help. In working with them to find a solution, we settled on trying out the assistance of a close neighbor who owed them a favor and was always asking if there was anything she could do to help. Fortunately, this neighbor lady was someone who enjoyed cleaning and organizing, and had a helpful and friendly attitude. She said she would love to come on a weekly basis for 4 hours for cleaning and clearing. This worked out great, and everyone enjoyed it. The neighbor felt she was finally able to pay back Dottie and Bud for the many years she had been allowed to use one of their sheds for storage. Dottie had a weekly time of visits, and felt great having her home cleaned. Bud had four hours of doing whatever he wanted, and felt his wife was in good hands so he could take off.

As time went on, the frequency of the visits decreased to every two weeks; then once a month. We made a few medication adjustments, and continued to put them in med sets to last a month. She did a stellar job of taking them once they were organized. She always arrived at her visits to the center early, and always with Bud. They had a close relationship, and after her mobility limitations due to the stroke, he compensated by being more helpful by wheeling her around in a wheelchair or ensuring her walker was nearby. She acted as interpreter for him, listening patiently with a gentle smile while he talked, then sharing what he was trying to communicate. It was quite cute, unless he was longwinded and I was short on time.

In the three years I cared for her, she stayed out of the hospital and was stable. Their life seemed to be quite comfortable and settled during that time. Then one Fall day I got a phone call from the kind neighbor who said Dottie had passed away in her sleep. I was sad, but thankful that she died peacefully at home. I tried several times to reach Bud by phone without success, but I was able to leave a message for him. I was sure he was having a difficult time without his helpmate. He called me several months later, and I was able to hear the heartache in his voice.

He stopped by the center about a year later. I was walking through the waiting room, and he was sitting there, patiently waiting for me to pass through. I have no idea how long he had been there. His eyes lit up when he saw me, and he jumped out of his chair with open arms. I gave him a hearty hug, and asked if he wanted to talk for a minute, so he followed me to the exam room and sat down. He was able, in his odd and halting way of talking, to thank me for all the help for his beloved wife Dottie. As he spoke, a small tear trickled down his rough, unshaven cheek. I teared up, patted his hand, and said he and Dottie had been a blessing to me, and I was honored to have been the trusted caregiver for the time allotted.

When Patients are Sandwich Caregivers

Sometimes a patient isn't the only one in need. There are times when the patient we are caring for is in turn caring for a loved one. Yes, the assumption is that this is an aging parent, but sometimes it is an offspring.

In the case of Carol, in addition to being a patient in great need of care, she also was the caregiver for not only a parent, and not only one son, but TWO!

A Tiny Strength

Carol came to the center after many hospitalizations for heart failure, stroke, and respiratory distress. After her stroke she had a decrease in her ability to swallow, and had a feeding tube inserted into her stomach and was told not to eat. She hated the feeding tube, and would try to eat or drink small amounts at home, with variable success. Sometimes she was able to tolerate it without problems, but other times she would aspirate, choke and end up with difficulty breathing. Usually she ended up in the hospital, having a tube inserted into her air passage and being hooked up to a breathing machine. Sometimes she developed aspiration pneumonia, and had to spend time in the ICU for a week or so.

She had a limited support system. She was divorced and had moved in to the house she was raised in to help her aging mom. This was a challenge because Carol not only had difficulty swallowing from her stroke, but her equilibrium was off enough to cause constant unsteadiness, with some stumbling and falling. She was unwilling to use a walker or even a cane. Besides her aging mom, she had two sons that lived on the property. According to Carol, one was sweet, but a useless alcoholic. He lived in a trailer on the property. The other son was aggressive and self-centered and had moved into granny's house without the consent of his mom or grandmother. He was also dealing drugs, or so Carol thought. Carol had many friends at church, where she and her mother had prepared weekly flower arrangements. None of those friends were confidants or close enough for Carol to share some of her difficulties. In reality, they likely would have been a big support in practical and emotional ways, but Carol did not want to burden them.

I had many concerns. She had been very unstable physically, with many hospitalizations. However, when discharged, she dove right back in to her many home responsibilities. Her self-care suffered because she was more focused on caring for her mom and trying her best to keep a safe and harmonious environment despite her one son. She also disliked the feeding tube. She found it uncomfortable, missed the eating and drinking, and did not like the tube feeding formula because it caused pretty severe diarrhea. Overall, she was having a hard time coping. Despite this, one would never know this from looking at her. She was lovely, tiny at about 100 pounds, always neatly dressed with matching colors, nice makeup and lovely hair. She never complained. When speaking about some of the struggles in her life she talked factually and kindly. Her main concern was her mother.

In stabilizing Carol, the technique that was useful was to work on things that would help her to be better able to care for her mom. Because that was difficult when she was not well or in the hospital, we set a goal of trying to keep her home so she could best help her mother. We set up a schedule and plan for which direction to head.

First, we had to set up a workable schedule for her medications, which we did by maximizing once-a-day dosing instead of twice a day. Then I helped her with a med set because she did not have the strength and agility in her hands to open the bottles; this had previously led to her not taking her medications. This thrilled her, because it had been causing great frustration. Then we worked out a system for the feeding tube. She found it difficult during her busy day to manually do multiple feedings, so we managed to work with her primary doctor to get a nighttime automatic system ordered and set up. We also arranged an appointment at the wound center because the area around the tube was having painful skin breakdown and rashes. The type of formula was changed to one less likely to cause gastric distress and diarrhea. In a short time her life dramatically improved!

I had a scary incident during one of her visits to the center. Her son had brought her in, and was sprawled out half asleep in the waiting room. I wanted him to join us for part of the visit so I could try to get his assistance in opening his mom's medication bottles. That way we could lengthen out her visits into the center. I also wanted to see if he could help his tiny mom when his grandmother needed assistance with some things that took strength. These seemed like simple enough tasks that a young man could help with, without too much inconvenience, especially since he was living there rent free!

I started by telling him how much better his mother was, and how she was staying out of the hospital. Carol was on the exam table, which I had put into a chair position. I was in the corner to her side, and her son was on a chair between the door and us. Big mistake! I gently asked if he would be willing to lend some small assistance to his mom and grandma, and he went into a rage! He stood up, with clenched fists and flushed face, and sputtered, "I do nothing but help them! Why do you think I moved back in?! They always need one thing or another! You think I do nothing for them! Well you are wrong, and I am out of here! I will never bring her back here again!!!!" Then he stormed out! I was glad to see him go because I am not comfortable with anger or aggression, and I did not want either Carol or me to be attacked. I was very concerned about her and did not want her to leave with him. She assured me he would be waiting in the car, and would be apologetic and quiet, and that he never touched her or her mom. She asked me not to call the authorities because she did not have bail money if he was thrown into jail. She told me things would be okay, and she could get by without his help. I never saw him again, and she never talked about him again. I watched for bruises or other signs of abuse, but never saw any. She continued to be prompt at all of her visits to the center, well put together, always pleasant and optimistic.

We encouraged her to accept hospice care for her mother, which she did. It was a big burden off of her because aids came daily to the house. There were also social workers, nurses and chaplains helping; Carol had a team of helpers. One of the aids also helped Carol remove the caps from her medication bottles, so this was a helpful solution to that problem. The automatic feeding tube greatly helped, and after about 6 months Carol was able to pass an evaluation that showed her swallowing had improved to the point she could have the tube removed and return to eating and drinking honey think liquids. She was thrilled!

Her sweet mother passed away several months later, and Carol was sad but relieved. A few months later I received a call from her son (the one who had stormed out of the exam room), sobbing and barely able to talk. He told me he had found his mom in her bedroom, unresponsive. He had called the medics, who were unable to resuscitate her. He shared he wished he had been a better son, and had been more helpful to her. Poor guy, he was so full of regrets and remorse. I allowed him to talk, then gently said he likely did the best he could at the time, and that it was never too late to improve his life. I told him that his mom would like for him to do that. He seemed to be encouraged from those words, and said he would do best. I never saw him again, but I hope he did change. He was a scary guy.

A Crooked Path to Recovery

Sometimes the journey from illness and disease is a straight path, but often it is a serpentine path leading this way and that. In other cases, it actually goes backwards for a while.

It is at times like these that the full resources of the patient's healthcare team must band together.

A Gentle Giant

Wade looked scary, but he was very sweet and sensitive. He was about 6'6", 400 pounds, with a pale complexion and flowing red hair past his shoulders. He had had a difficult hospitalization, with a new diagnosis of high blood pressure and heart failure due to a rapid, irregular heart rhythm called atrial fibrillation. He was also an alcoholic, used to consuming a case of beer and a liter of wine daily prior to his hospitalization. He had not had a drink since.

He had never married and lived by himself a few blocks from the hospital. His supportive mother accompanied him to the initial visit. She was kind, trim, and quite bright. She was especially interested in the dietary education because she was a nutritionist. She shared that she hoped this was a turning point for Wade, and that he would improve his eating and abstain from alcohol. He shared that he was motivated to do both.

As the weeks went by, he gradually improved and became stronger. He was bright and motivated. He took his medications as prescribed, and tried to weigh himself consistently at the cargo scale of the hospital. His weight was too high for a home scale. He tried to improve his eating with lower sodium foods, but he continued to eat excessive amounts. I encouraged him along, and did not push him too hard on weight loss at this time, because he had stopped drinking and was taking his meds. The obesity would be addressed at a later time.

As he got stronger, we worked out a walking program. It had to work out with his 90 year old neighbor's schedule, because she had to put on his shoes and socks (his obesity prevented him from bending over to do it himself). Wade started with 5 minutes a day for the first week, then he tried to increase it a minute a week. This seemed to work out pretty well for him, and he said it increased his energy and helped to tone him up a bit. We also hoped that it would help with a slow, steady weight loss. He was motivated and disciplined with this until his mom developed serious health problems, and passed away shortly thereafter. Wade's life went for a bit of a tailspin there, because his mother had been the glue that held his family together. She had also made his clothes, bought his medications, and gave him money for food. He made a living from a home-based business, but it sounded like his earnings did not pay all his expenses. Unfortunately, his father and other family members did not step forward to help out.

He did not go back to drinking alcohol during this stressful time, but he did get off schedule a bit with medications. Fortunately, he discussed this with us, and we were able to help. We had applied for and received a grant we used for medications for those we deemed unable to afford them, so we were able to get him a monthly supply of the medications. We supplemented with sample packs from the pharmaceutical companies, and had the social worker help with applications for discounted medications from the drug companies. This helped to return him to consistent medication administration.

He was sad, lonely, and depressed. His mother had been an excellent support for him in many ways, and he really missed that. He was quite socially isolated, and his elderly neighbor was the only one he saw during the week. His visits to our center were now monthly. He agreed to see a behavioral health psychiatrist who was quite helpful for getting him through his grief and depression.

A few years went by in a relatively stable manner for Wade. He stayed out of the hospital, took fairly good care of himself, with the exception of a bit of a weight gain. Then one day, while shopping, he gave into the temptation of buying some vodka. "Just one bottle," he said to himself. Well, one drink became two, and then we was drinking a fifth of vodka a day. His health deteriorated, and he had a respiratory arrest, but the medics found him in time and he was brought to the hospital. Critically ill, on life support, with a 40 day hospitalization!

When he finally returned home after a prolonged hospitalization, and time at a skilled nursing facility, it took him a long time to return to feeling as well as he had before he started drinking again. But slowly, steadily he progressed, week by week getting stronger. Although he lacked the loving support of his mother, he still had the neighbor. He had also established friendships via his home computer, which was nice for him since he was home most of the time. He enjoyed this very much, and looked forward to correspondence throughout the day and into the night. He returned to his hopeful and appreciative self, and had others encouraging him towards improved health.

The Way it is Supposed to End

It is fitting to end my stories with a success story.

In healthcare, we do not claim to provide our patients with eternal life. We all know that our days on earth are numbered from the day of our birth. Instead, our intent is to provide the care needed to allow people to lead healthy lives with the lifestyle of their choosing.

I only wish I could tell such a story about all my patients.

A Political Dynamo

James was one of my first patients, and I cared for him until his death at a conference after he delivered a moving, inspiring fundraising speech for one of our state's politicians. That was an appropriate way for him to spend his final time on earth, because he was being productive at supporting a cause he believed in. Also, because he always said; "I want to die with my shoes on," which he did.

Looking at him the first time I met him, it was difficult to envision him as a strong leader and an excellent speaker. He looked frail, in a wheelchair pushed by his little, but hardy wife. His voice was weak, with frequent pauses; but his words were eloquent and thoughtful. He had been in the hospital for about two weeks, with a new diagnosis of heart failure due to coronary artery disease. He was now home, in the care of his wife, and was somewhat discouraged with his diagnosis and extreme weakness. He and his wife were also extremely motivated and very bright. They seemed to hang on every word of explanations and encouragement I offered. It is important to be optimistic and encouraging in heart failure management, or any chronic disease. These patients are quite ill, and need someone to partner with them and move them physically and emotionally towards improved health.

I usually do not make any medication changes at the initial visit to the center, however James needed an extra diuretic to ease his shortness of breath and leg swelling. He had not been monitoring these things at home because he did not receive instructions while in the hospital about the importance of monitoring these things. Perhaps he did receive it, but was too ill or overwhelmed to retain it, which is sometimes the case. Repetition and consistency is essential in the education of chronic disease.

On the day of his initial visit, he and his wife were like sponges soaking up the information. I sent him home with a scale and a chart to monitor his daily weight and signs and symptoms, as well as a medication list and instructions to increase his diuretic. Then an appointment was made to see him the following week.

I saw him weekly for months and saw him stabilize and improve. He became quite feisty and talkative, and would become animated when describing his life. He was in his 80s, but would still go to the office at a company he started in order to work a few hours a day. He was thrilled he was feeling well enough to continue to do that.

One day, halfway through his visit to see me, he said "Nancy, I have a concern." I sat down, looked at him and said "Would you like to share it?" He paused, looked at me intently, and quietly said, "I am concerned I will get too healthy to come to see you." I smiled, held his hand, and said "James, no need to be concerned about that, because the door of the center is always open to you." A smile of relief spread across his face. His wife smiled behind him, and the anxiety seemed to flow out of the room.

Performance Outcomes

We called our clinic The Cardiac Enhancement Center. Patients and their loved ones usually told us they liked that name. They said it was positive and hopeful, in contrast to Heart Failure Center.

We were given the freedom to set it up from the ground up as we wanted, or more importantly, in a manner that best met the patients' needs. The medical director was an excellent cardiologist with a specialty in heart failure management and was great to work with. He was bright and innovative. He had also worked with some excellent nurse practitioners, so he was used to the level of knowledge and expertise they had. Basically, I was, as a nurse practitioner, able to set up an efficient, cost-effective, patient-focused center. Our goal was to significantly improve the quality of life for our patients, and to do so in a cost-effective manner.

We were a hospital-based, outpatient center, located in a separate building from the hospital. We shared the lobby and some administrative assistance with two other hospital-based centers, one for anticoagulation and one for lipid management. Both were staffed by warm, caring, cooperative, and respectful professionals. Our center started small, with just a part-time nurse practitioner (me) working 30 hours a week, and a medical director who was there for guidance and support who I met with for an hour or so once a week. The foundational work was immense: ordering supplies, creating forms, writing protocols, and planning the specifics of the management of patients. I had worked in cardiology all of my professional life, from critical cares to cardiac rehab, patient and family education, as well as education of nurses at the college level. Before I was asked to start this center, I was in a practice at a nearby hospital with a cardiology group caring for patients in the hospital and the clinic.

During my years of caring for patients with heart problems, my favorites were those with heart failure. They were the sickest, and usually had multiple other health problems like diabetes, coronary artery disease, high blood pressure, kidney problem, and depression. It was also the population that was in the hospital most frequently. Once in the hospital, there was a very high chance that this same patient would have to return to the hospital within 30 days of discharge. Nationwide, their care was often fragmented, with a different provider seeing them in the emergency room, caring for them in the hospital, and caring for them once leaving the hospital. Each provider frequently adjusted, stopped or changed medications. Fragmented care combined with complex illnesses is a horrible combination. Daily monitoring and home self-management is also essential, and those without a good support system at home are at higher risk of going to the hospital. The burden of care for patients, families, the health care system, hospitals and society is tremendous.

In 2012, it is estimated there were over 5 million people with a diagnosis of heart failure, and the annual death rate is 300,000 a year nationally. It is increasing annually, with a projected prevalence of 10 million patients in the U.S. by 2037. Heart failure is the leading cause of hospitalizations in adults age 65 and older, and hospitalizations for heart failure are associated with increased morbidity and mortality. Heart failure results in over 1,000,000 admissions when it is the primary diagnosis, and twice that many when it is a secondary diagnosis. Either way, heart failure results in 6.5 million hospital days per year.

Nationally, about one quarter of the patients have to return to the hospital within a month. The annual re-admission a year rakes up more than $17 billion in annual Medicare costs. Many of these re-admissions are avoidable, with a range of expert opinion citing from 40% to 75% of them. This situation creates a tremendous cost to society, with an average hospitalization in 2012 costing about $8,000. Almost 2/3 of the costs of heart failure are due to hospital care. Heart failure is the reason for 12 to 15 million clinic visits a year.

As a healthcare system, we are reacting to heart failure, not treating it.

When the data at our particular hospital was evaluated before the center was established, a chart review showed almost 40% of patients admitted with heart failure were re-admitted within a month. The follow-up care was inconsistent. We were ready to improve this situation, for our patient satisfaction and safety as well as the fiscal management of the hospital.

For starters, it was important to shift the care to the outpatient arena, which could be a place with increased continuity. A center had to be patient and family focused, affirming, accessible, and responsive to needs. Our care needed to use evidence-based knowledge of how to stabilize and improve heart failure along with the art of empowering patients and families to be involved in their care and to take the medications and treatment prescribed. A team approach was mandatory because each professional had their various gifts, abilities, and expertise.

One of the foundational steps in setting up the center was to determine who was involved in the care of these patients throughout the continuum of health care, then to set up an avenue for communication and education. This would include patients; families; nurses from the hospital's 24/7 call center; emergency room doctors and nurses; health care providers in the hospital; primary care providers; social workers; nutritionists; cardiac rehab nurses and exercise physiologists; quality improvement experts; staff from the skilled nursing centers and senior centers; and hospice and palliative care social workers and nurses. Quite a team! As I met and networked with some of these people, the list narrowed to specific faces of those who had an interest in meeting regularly to strive to improve the care of patients with heart failure. A team began to form!

We started to meet monthly for an efficient, action-packed, productive hour. I chaired it, had a planned agenda for each meeting, and started and finished promptly. It consisted of presentations pertinent to the care of these patients, changing policies, addressing and solving problems, and working as a team on care improvement. The team was professionals from The Cardiac Enhancement Center, patient advisors, the medical director, RNs from the 24/7 call center, the quality improvement director, a representative from cardiac rehab, the director of nursing from a major skilled nursing facility, a nutritionist, social workers and nurses involved in discharge planning, nurse managers from the units caring for these patients, and hospice and palliative care nurse managers.

Simultaneously, there was a need to meet with the doctors and nurse practitioners in the area to find out what their needs were, and how a center for heart failure management could augment the care they provided. This was important, since patients were referred to the center for care. The medical director and I provided opportunities for them to meet with us in person, or give us their opinions via surveys and questionnaires. This was very valuable because we wanted to provide a center that would augment the care they provided, not steal patients away from them.

An assessment of the care and education patients received in the hospital was done. It showed the care could be streamlined and simplified, so we began to formulate a standardized order set to be used when a patient with heart failure was admitted. We also wanted to increase the knowledge level of the nurses and assistants caring for these patients, so educational sessions were formulated. During this time, over 400 caregivers attended a class on heart failure signs and symptoms and patient care. A review of patient education on the topic showed deficits, so a team worked on compiling some simple but effective tools. This also included the documentation of the education.

After compiling a packet of education materials for patients and families on heart failure management, a system was developed to get it into the hands of those who needed it. The standard of care was that every bedside nurse was responsible for patient education, so we provided the packets on each unit and informed the staff of their availability. When this was first done, the majority of patients did not receive the packet or verbal teaching. Various methods were tried to increase this, but none were effective. Therefore, an efficient and streamlined way to get this done was to have a core of motivated nurses who enjoyed patient education and were accountable for this in their job description. This core was a few nurses from our 24/7 hospital call center who were trained and motivated to identify the target patient population, initiate the education, document the education, and then do the follow- up phone calls at discharge. The call occurred a few days after discharge, then weekly for a month. The frequency was varied depending on the need. They also assessed the support system at home from the information they were able to gather while the patient was in the hospital. They did an excellent job and were an essential part of the team involved in providing high quality care for heart failure patients. Eventually, they even began to schedule the follow up appointments for these patients. These nurses, who we entitled "Heart Failure Resource Nurses," were an essential link between the in-patient care and the out-patient center. Most patients reported feeling cared about and greatly helped by their services.

A review of the literature was also done in order to look at various models of heart failure centers. We wanted to start a state-of- the-art, innovative center that provided the best possible care for patients and families in a cost-effective, efficient manner. The Institute of Healthcare Improvement cites three aims (called The Triple Aim) of patient care:

1. *Improving the patient experience of care*
2. *Improving the health of the population*
3. *Reducing cost*

Our goals were consistent with this. Because we were starting from the ground up, and starting small, we were able to pick and choose from various models and set up a center that would work for us and the community. It was essential that we had an excellent, innovative, and supportive CEO of the hospital during the initial stages, and for the majority of the years we did this.

In a chronic disease like heart failure, it is essential to allow enough time to adequately evaluate all aspects of each patient. This includes a comprehensive health history, medications, allergies, past medical and surgical history, and psychosocial situation. The psycho-social evaluation is important because it addresses the support system, and any physical, psychological, financial, educational, or cultural barrier to improved health. To allow adequate time, the health records were reviewed and a comprehensive problem list was compiled prior to the patient's initial visit, and 90 minutes were allocated for the one-on-one time with the patient and family member(s) (or close friend). The return visits to the center ranged from 30 to 60 minutes. All of the time was with a cardiology nurse practitioner, either me or those we hired after a few years. We did not have nursing assistants. We did have administrative assistance, however, to help with the enormous paper pile as the patient load grew. They also helped to maintain the friendly, patient-focused care we wanted to provide at all times.

After every patient visit to the center we dictated a comprehensive note for both the initial visit as well as the progress notes for the ongoing visits. These were sent to all the other providers who were involved in the care of each patient. They were essential in keeping everyone informed and updated on the patient's progress and medication changes. At each visit the patient was sent home with an accurate, updated medication list. We also usually made out a "to do" list for them. We found these to be essential in providing safe, continuity of care.

With a chronic disease like heart failure, we thought it was essential to see patients frequently. This usually consisted of every 2 weeks as we were initiating and adjusting medications, as well as evaluating the person's motivation and ability to manage their care at home. Once their medications were stabilized and they were improved, we lengthened it out to every month. Even with a person who was extremely stable, we continued to see them every three months. Inevitably, things were picked up at each visit, and adjustments were made. Early interventions on an outpatient basis have been shown to decrease hospitalizations, and we consistently found that to be true at our center.

Because the type of heart failure management at our Cardiac Enhancement Center was a new model, we thought it would be important to keep track of outcomes to see if we were making a positive impact. We looked at the Minnesota Living with Heart Failure Questionnaire, the 6 minute walk test, and the Beck Depression at the initial visit to the center, and at 3 months. The results showed remarkable improvement, the details of which will be provided on the following pages. We also wanted to keep track of admissions to the hospital, but for the first several years our hospital records were not able to obtain that information. I tried to do it myself, however I found there were times I was not made aware of patient's admissions so it was falsely low. The last few years the EMR were set up to obtain the information, and it showed readmission results well below the national average. So the outcomes showed the quality of life improved and the re-admission rate decreased. We also obtained patient satisfaction results through standardized questions via the call center which showed excellence in all areas. It showed we were quite successful in all areas.

We were a high touch, low technology center. The only equipment we had at the center was a large, sturdy scale that went to 1000 pounds, manual blood pressure cuffs, oxygen saturation finger monitors, a machine to check transthoracic impedance called a BioZ, and excellent stethoscopes. We also had syringes to administer influenza and pneumococcal vaccinations, which we would do routinely for our patients. We thought it was important to provide this protection, because getting pneumonia and influenza can exacerbate heart failure and push these fragile patients into the hospital. The center was also filled with abundant education material, such as cardiac risk factor reduction and heart disease, heart healthy eating and low sodium recipes, depression and anxiety, and information about atrial fibrillation, high blood pressure, kidney disease, gout, and sleep apnea.

Although we were a small cost center, with 2 nurse practitioners and 2 administrative assistants, plus a medical director who charged us for hourly services (maybe 4 to 10 hours a month), we were busy but not a big money maker for the hospital. We saw from 6 to 16 patients a day, mostly Medicare, which does not reimburse much. We also had many DSHS patients, and King County Project Access patients who did not pay anything. We barely broke even, however our philosophy was that by stabilizing patients on an outpatient basis and keeping them out of the hospital we were saving the hospital money (nationwide, a hospital loses close to $2000 per hospitalization for a heart failure patient, because the reimbursement is less than the cost to care for *them). Also it was the right thing to do for patients and families and the greater good for society. It was an effective model that can be replicated, and likely similar models will be utilized by many places around the country for chronic disease management in the future.*

Patient Improvements

Between spring 2003 and 2012, over 1000 patients were referred to the center for heart failure management. The majority of the referrals came from cardiologists, with about 15% coming from primary care providers. When we looked at this closely we found this was because, in our area, most of those with heart disease were under cardiology care. The age range of patients was from 19 to 104, with the average age of 69. 41% were woman and 59% men.

Common co-morbidities consisted of 38% with diabetes, 19% with anemia, 30% with kidney impairment, and 34% with depression. We found the list of patient problems ranged from a low of 4 to a high of 23, with an average of 9 current problems or co-morbidities. In other words, there were complicated patients.

Our quality outcomes showed improvement, with an average as below:

- *Minnesota Living with Heart Failure improved by 23%.*
- *6 minute walk test improved by 32%.*
- *Beck Depression or PHQ9 improved by 11%.*
- *The hearts function, as measured by the Ejection fraction, improved by 21.5 points (for those with systolic heart failure).*
- *97% of our patients were on beta blockers*
- *92% of our patients were on ACE Inhibitors or ARBS*

- *Our re-admission rate in 2010 was down to 12.4% (about half of the national average).*

These improvements in outcomes showed that the model of care we set up was successful. We improved the quality of life for patients, as showed by the Minnesota Living with Heart Failure questionnaire, there was also improvement in the 6 minute walk test, and patients were less depressed. This is quite remarkable, considering heart failure is a chronic, progressive disease state. We also had shown our Cardiac Enhancement Center was consistent with The Institute of Medicine's Six Aims for Care, which are:

1. *Safe*
2. *Effective*
3. *Patient centered*
4. *Timely*
5. *Efficient*
6. *Equitable*

The majority of our patients were also on the evidence-based medicine, and were staying out of the hospital in a much greater number than those treated in conventional manners nationwide. It was also a cost-effective model, because we were optimally managing patients on an outpatient basis, instead of the net money loss at hospitalization. True, any management of Medicare patients is not a big money maker because the reimbursement is a fraction of the cost to care for them whether it is outpatient or inpatient; however it is much less expensive on an outpatient basis as compared to hospitalization.

In summary, healthcare is a science, but it is far more about relationships. It is an art. My experiences would suggest that there is great benefit for all parties when more attention is paid to the art of healthcare when applying the science of healthcare. A relationship-based approach can produce far more positive outcomes, can produce far more content patients and families, and at least in the case of this one healthcare provider, it provided incredible rewards in the form of memories that will last the rest of my life.